TESTOSTERONE

THE TESTOSTERONE BIBLE

BOOST TESTOSTERONE NATURALLY FOR WEIGHT LOSS, MUSCLE BUILDING, LIBIDO & ERECTILE DYSFUNCTION

CHASE WILLIAMS

© 2016

COPYRIGHT NOTICE

DISCLAIMER

Although the author and publisher have made every effort to ensure that the information in this book was correct at press time, the author and publisher do not assume and hereby disclaim any liability to any party for any loss, damage, or disruption caused by errors or omissions, whether such errors or omissions result from negligence, accident, or any other cause.

TABLE OF CONTENTS

INTRODUCTION

If you are reading this book, chances are you may have signs that your testosterone level is low, such as having low libido (or sex drive), lack of energy, an increase in fat production or a decrease in muscle mass. Perhaps you may have read some articles on testosterone and have been wondering if perhaps you might be able to increase your testosterone to increase your own sex drive. Or you may have found out from your doctor that you do, indeed, have low testosterone and you may be wondering just what testosterone is and whether Testosterone Replacement Therapy is necessary or if there is any way you can possibly increase your testosterone naturally.

Either way, this book is for you. While both men and women produce testosterone, this hormone is much more important (and much more prevalent) in men than in women and I am making the supposition that you are a man, (or a woman who is reading it to help her man), if you are reading this book. With that in mind, most of the information contained herein is written for men to increase their testosterone, but women may also find it helpful and beneficial as well in some way.

According to recent statistics as many as one in four men suffer from low testosterone and many of them do not even realize that this is the problem. In this book you will learn that testosterone levels tend to diminish as we get older, and this may affect our virility, drive, manliness and overall health (sexual and otherwise).

The first couple of chapters are kept succinct and to the point so you can gain a working knowledge of Testosterone without having to be burdened with a plethora of scientific and medical terminology. You will learn that once your testosterone level drops you may experience mood changes such as irritability and depression), fatigue, low sex drive, erectile dysfunction, reduced muscle mass, increased fat, and host of other problems that affects your quality of life.

You will be given a brief overview of what exactly testosterone is and how testosterone is produced in the body. We will go on to explain how you can get your testosterone tested, what you can expect from the tests, and the various Testosterone Replacement Treatment options available.

The rest of this book is really the meat and potatoes (so to speak) of the book, in that you will find out how you can increase your testosterone level naturally, through several different "lifestyle changes" that you can put to work immediately. While these changes are (on the surface) quite simple, and easy to institute, when instituted they are guaranteed to raise your testosterone levels, while increasing your energy, vitality and the very quality of your life.

While you may be wondering how much you can actually get out of such a short book, you'll find that after reading this book and putting those principles outlined in this book into practice, it may be the most important book you have ever picked up. In fact, if you do put these principles into practice you will find that not only will your sex live be dramatically enhanced, but you will be healthier and happier than you may have ever realized you could feel. You will have more energy and more vitality that you might have thought possible, and you will increase your mental and physical health to unforeseen levels in a very short time.

As I tell many of my readers, while this book is really a life changer, simply reading it won't really do much at all for you, other than give you insight into how much better you can be. You MUST put these principles and methods into effect, in order for them to work for you. I can tell you with 100% certainty, however, that by taking that step and putting these methods to work for you, you will not be sorry. You will become the man you may have once been, or may never have been. You will become more confident in yourself and your abilities. You will have peace of mind and vitality of life that will make you feel like a new man.

All of this isn't just hype, though it is meant to motivate you and make you realize the importance of not only reading this but really going through with the plans, procedures and methods outlined. Once you have finished reading this book, you may want to read it again, and maybe a third time just to make sure you understand what you can achieve. Even before you finish you may find yourself putting many of the principles into action and you may find yourself already becoming more like the man you know you can be. So take the first step and start with that first chapter, then read on until you find the secret to improving your life by increasing your testosterone to peak levels.

Go ahead, turn to that first page... and start your journey to becoming the new you! As the saying goes, a journey of a thousand miles begins with a single step. You have already taken the first step by picking up this book... now begins your journey... enjoy the new life you are about to discover!

CHAPTER 1: WHAT IS TESTOSTERONE? (A BRIEF DESCRIPTION)

While most people have heard of testosterone, when it comes to defining it it's a safe bet to say most people have little to no idea what testosterone actually is. It may be known that testosterone is a hormone important in sexual development and sexual activity, but for most people that's as far as the knowledge goes. In reality, testosterone plays a much larger role in our health and well being and a better understanding of what it is and how it works will go a long way in understanding why a healthy level of testosterone is imperative in order to maintain our health.

While testosterone is considered a male sex hormone, women also produce testosterone, albeit on a much lower level than men. The NIH (National Institute of Health) categorizes testosterone as the single most important male hormone as it is instrumental in the development of sex organs even before birth and is also involved in the development of secondary sexual characteristics during puberty; such as penis and testes size, growth of body and facial hair and deepening of voice. It is also important for the production of sperm, distribution of fat, production of red blood cells and conditioning of muscle strength.

Testosterone is classified as an androgen, also called steroids or anabolic steroids. It is manufactured in the testes in man and in the ovaries in women. The production of testosterone is regulated by hormones that the brain releases, in particular the hormone production is signaled by the hypothalamus and pituitary gland. These produce signals for hormonal production, which travel throughout the bloodstream and activate sexual organs in men as well as women. The hypothalamus tells the pituitary gland how much testosterone it needs to produce, which is then passed on to the testes in men or the ovaries and adrenal glands in women. The levels of testosterone in women are around 1/10 to 1/20th of that produced in man.

Testosterone is produced in men via interstitial cells or Leydig cells. The cells are located between the seminiferous tubules of the testis (responsible for producing sperm) . These Leydig cells are responsible for the secretion of testosterone as well as androstenedione and dehydroepiandrosterone (DHEA). When Leydig cells are exposed to Luteneizing Hormone (LH), they will produce androgens, which includes testosterone. Luteneizing Hormone is a glycoprotein, a protein connected to a sugar moiety. This is one of two gonadotropins, with the other protein being the Follicle Stimulating Hormone or FSH. LH and FSH work in conjunction to stimulate cells of the follicle in order to produce estrogen. The Leydig cells in male testes respond to the Luteneizing Hormone by producing testosterone.

The testosterone level in boys is usually very low before puberty. After puberty hits, the levels increase until it reaches it's highest level around age 40, when it generally begins to gradually decrease. As a matter of fact, it's been estimated that around 4 out of 10 men aged 45+ are suffering from low testosterone.

Often Low testosterone is blamed for erectile dysfunction, however low testosterone does not necessarily impair the actual ability to get an erection. Low testosterone usually has more to do with low sex drive and low libido. Erectile dysfunction can have many different causes, such as high cholesterol and high blood pressure or psychological causes, such as depression and anxiety disorders. However, erections are dependent on testosterone and many chronic conditions caused by low testosterone also play a large role in erectile dysfunction. We will examine many of these conditions in the next chapter, but you should be aware that if you are suffering from erectile dysfunction, simply improving your testosterone level may not help. Only your doctor can tell you whether you are suffering from low testosterone (aka Low T count), and whether it is contributing to erectile dysfunction, or whether the dysfunction is linked to a low sex drive, rather than the ability to retain an erection.

In any case if your testosterone level is low, you may find yourself experiencing many different symptoms, including erectile dysfunction or weak erections, low sex drive, low energy, and a host of other problems, which we will be discussing in the next chapter. While these symptoms may actually be due to some other issue, chances are if you have 3 or more of these symptoms you are suffering from low testosterone and will want to begin a program of increasing your testosterone as quickly as possible.

CHAPTER 2: LOW TESTOSTERONE TESTING & TREATING

As discussed briefly in the preceding chapter, many men over the age of 40 may be suffering from low testosterone. Some of the symptoms of "Low T count" includes:

- Low Sex Drive or Low Libido

- Fatigue

- Unexplainable Weight Gain (especially around the waist)

- Problems concentrating or focusing

- Depression

- Irritability

- Hair Loss

- Changes in the size of the testicles

While testosterone levels can vary quite a bit, from hour to hour (and even minute to minute) and between individuals, a healthy level of testosterone usually falls around 500 to 700 ng/dL (nanograms per deciliter). The lower limit usually falls around 300 ng/DL and the upper limit about 800 ng/dL. There are many different conditions that may contribute to a low testosterone level, aside from aging, such as:

- Testicular injury

- Testicular Cancer

- HIV/AIDS

- Obesity

- Type 2 diabetes

- Hormone disorders

- Some types of infections

- Several different medications

- Genetic Conditions

In many cases, it's desirable to find the root cause of the low T count, and treat this first, rather than simply trying to increase the testosterone level through Testosterone Replacement Therapies. Often, by addressing the underlying cause, the testosterone level will increase automatically.

Sometimes, however, the actual cause of these conditions is directly related to low testosterone levels and increasing the testosterone levels will dramatically improve or cure the condition. Often it is nearly impossible to separate the cause and condition. For instance, it's been noted that obesity can cause low testosterone levels while it's also noted that low testosterone levels may cause obesity. There will be some who find that Testosterone Replacement Therapy (TRT) actually helps them lose weight, whereas others may find their weight completely unaffected by TRT. In any case, the chapters following this may help to increase those conditions even if Testosterone Replacement Therapy is not indicated... but let's not get ahead of ourselves.

As the medical field is learning more about low testosterone and the many effects it can entail, we are seeing more doctors looking at Low Testosterone as the root, rather as one of the effects of things such as diabetes, depression, heart disease and high blood pressure. Doctors are now taking Low Testosterone much more seriously than ever before, where once upon a time, doctors only looked at testosterone levels when patients complained about their sex drive or their inability to retain erections.

Normally, testosterone testing is ordered for men with andropause (male menopause) or hypogonadism (inability to produce androgen (testosterone)). While testosterone levels in men do drop as they age, this is not considered hypogonadism and the FDA does not recommend Testosterone Replacement Therapy for low testosterone caused by aging.

However, many doctors are now ordering blood tests for testosterone levels as a standard practice when dealing with most of the preceding peripheral issues. It is now advisable, especially if you are over 40, to get your testosterone checked regularly, even if you are having no symptoms. Low testosterone levels can also lead to a decrease in bone density, which means fragile bones that can break more easily. It's been shown that raising the testosterone level often helps bone density before it get's too low and bone-related problems (such as osteoporosis) arise.

As mentioned Testosterone levels rise and fall during the day, sometimes quite dramatically. Your doctor will probably want to check your testosterone level early in the morning, when the levels tend to be highest. He or she may also want to test your testosterone levels several times at different times of the day to get an idea of your average T count. So, don't be surprised if our doctor has you come in several times for these tests.

When measuring testosterone levels, it is very important to measure both the free testosterone as well as the total testosterone levels. When your doctor checks for testosterone levels he or she will look at three different aspects of testosterone. The first two parts are attached (or bound) to two proteins; Albumin and Sex Hormone Binding Globulin (SHBG). The third type is not bound to either of the proteins and is therefore classified as "free testosterone". Testosterone bound to albumin and free testosterone are referred to as "bioavailable testosterone", as these are easily used by the body.

Aside from testing the free and total testosterone levels in your body, estradiol tests are also needed to discover if the testosterone in your body is not being excessively converted to estrogen. High levels of estrogen in men can contribute to prostate cancer as well as heart disease and in some cases gynecomastia (breast enlargement). If your test reveal that your estrogen levels are too high, your doctor may also prescribe the use of aromatase inhibitors, such as Chrysin or Arimidex.

Other tests that may be considered include testing of the Luteinizing Hormone (LH), SHBG levels, DHEA and Dihydrotestosterone. Your medical practitioner may also do a complete blood workup that includes blood cell count and chemistry profile (liver, kidney, lipids, glucose, mineral, etc.).

Due to the increase in education and understanding of the way testosterone affects your overall health, doctors are more and more prone to testing for testosterone levels than previously. However, you really shouldn't wait for your doctor to suggest testing for testosterone, but take the initiative and request test yourself. Especially if you are finding your sex drive low, or you experiencing other symptoms (as listed above) that may be rooted in low testosterone. You shouldn't be embarrassed to ask your doctor to schedule testosterone tests, as it's not only about your libido, but your overall health can be greatly affected by low levels of Testosterone.

While there isn't a "magic" number where testosterone is considered "low", most halth care professionals consider testosterone levels under 300 ng/dL to be low, and if your testosterone level falls well below 300 (such as 200 or 150 ng/dL) your doctor may advise a Testosterone Replacement Therapy, such as a regular regimen of testosterone injections. There are also other treatment methods, such as a patch or gel you can apply regularly, to keep the testosterone levels up. Another treatment method that is fairly new are pellets that are placed under the skin of the buttocks. These testosterone pellets releases the testosterone slowly over a few months period.

While low testosterone is treatable through these methods, there are possible side effects to undergoing a Testosterone Replacement Therapy, such as an increase in acne, a decrease in testicle size, enlargement of breasts and/or other side effects. It's best to talk to your doctor to understand what other side effects you may experience from Testosterone Replacement Therapy.

Most doctors will tell you that Testosterone Replacement Therapy is fairly safe if the treatments are monitored closely. However, it should also be noted that there is some concern within the medical community about the relationship between Testosterone Replacement Therapy and prostate health. This treatment is, therefore, not advised for patients with prostate cancer. More recently, however, data available from the National Institute of Health suggests that high testosterone levels are not actually associated with increased risk of prostate cancer.

There has, unfortunately, been very little research into the effects of long term testosterone treatments to date. Most medical practitioners have seen very few (or no) side effects to treatment therapy, but as this type of therapy becomes more common, there may surface unforeseen long term effects. While short term use of testosterone replacement has been (so far) fairly benign and the results have been (for the most part) very encouraging, when testosterone therapy ceases, the levels of testosterone usually end up going back down. This means that, in order to keep up the testosterone levels, ongoing treatment is necessary.

The good news, however, is that there are other ways that you can increase your testosterone level naturally. These methods will require you to change your lifestyle and diet. In the preceding chapters we will cover the different lifestyle and dietary changes you can make that will help increase your testosterone; in conjunction with Testosterone Replacement Therapy or by themselves, depending on how low your testosterone level is and/or the severity of symptoms you may be having.

CHAPTER 3: NATURAL METHODS FOR INCREASING TESTOSTERONE LEVELS

There are many ways (aside from Testosterone Replacement Therapy) to boost your testosterone level naturally. In many cases, by keeping to a healthy lifestyle and diet, you can increase your testosterone (and lower your estrogen) levels. There are also many supplements that are helpful in increasing testosterone. If you find yourself suffering from low testosterone, before you engage in Testosterone Replacement Therapy, look at your overall lifestyle and you may find that by simply changing a few simple things, you can boost your testosterone, while also increasing your overall vitality.

SLEEP

One major contributor to low testosterone levels that can usually be changed easily is the amount of sleep you are getting. A lack of sleep can play havoc with many hormones and chemicals in your body, and can be highly detrimental to your testosterone level. Most healthcare professionals recommend at least 7 to 9 hours of sleep per night for most adults (including older adults). Of course, the amount of sleep required may change from individual to individual. For instance, some people may get along fine with only 6 hours of sleep at night, while others may require as much as 10 hours of sleep. The best way to gauge whether you are getting enough sleep is by examining how drowsy you feel during the day. If you are getting less than 7 hours of sleep, and are having trouble concentrating during the day, then it's a good idea to try to up your sleep time.If you want to know your peak sleep time, you can slowly increase the time you are asleep until you feel at your best during the day.

If you find you are not getting enough sleep at night, there are ways you can help yourself increase your sleep time, and by doing so, increase your overall health, vitality, and testosterone levels. Some things to keep in mind for optimizing your sleep are:

1. Go to sleep at the same time each night and awake at the same time. This helps to set your sleep cycle (circadian rhythm).

2. Avoid sleeping in, as this can throw your sleep cycle off. If you find you haven't gotten enough sleep, opt for a short nap in the afternoon to make up for the lost sleep.

3. Limit any naps to 15 or 20 minutes.

4. Make your sleeping area as comfortable as possible, adjusting the temperature so you are neither too hot or too cold.

5. Make sure your sleeping area is dark enough, if necessary install dark drapes or curtains. Your brain produces melatonin (a naturally occurring hormone) when it is dark, which tells your brain it's time to sleep.

6. Don't use your bed for other activities such as watching TV or reading, if possible. By using your bed ONLY for sleeping, you will train your brain (more or less) to recognize that bed means sleep, and you will find it much easier to fall asleep once your head hits the pillow.

7. Avoid eating large meals before bedtime; some people find that a small snack before bedtime is helpful, such as a bowl of granola or half a turkey sandwich. Just don't overdo it.

8. Limit caffeine. While you may have heard not to consume drinks with caffeine within a couple of hours of sleep, you may not realize caffeine can cause sleep problems even up to 12 hours after consumption, especially in those who are sensitive to caffeine.

9. Some people find that low-impact exercises such as yoga, foam rolling, and stretching exercises can help them fall asleep. But rigorous workouts should be avoided close to bedtime as your body temperature is raised, your metabolism speeds up and your body produces hormones that makes you more alert.

10. Regular vigorous exercises during the day can help many sleep problems, including sleep apnea and insomnia. However, it may take months of regular exercise regimen before the sleep benefits are noticeable.

These are just a few tips that can help you get the proper amount of sleep at night. If these don't seem to help you, you may be suffering from sleep apnea or some other sleep disorder, and it would be advisable to discuss your sleep problems with your doctor. Sometimes a sleep supplement such as melatonin can help you to adjust your sleep cycle. However, it is inadvisable to use any sleep inducing drugs or supplements over a long period of time as your body may become dependent on them. You should discuss with your doctor any supplement or any OTC sleep aid before taking them.

Exercise

A sedentary lifestyle is often a chief cause of low testosterone. If you spend most of your time sitting on the couch, watching TV or sitting in front of a computer, it is actually signalling your brain that it doesn't need to produce as much testosterone, as your muscles and bones do not require this hormone. On the other hand, if you spend time each day exercising, your brain will send out the signal that it needs more testosterone.Also, a lack of regular exercise may also lead to obesity, which affects the amount of testosterone your body produces.

If you aren't getting enough exercise now, you should try to gradually increase your physical activities throughout the day. One excellent way to increase your exercise is by simply taking a brisk afternoon walk, for about 20 minutes per day. You can gradually increase the time/distance as your body gets used to this new activity.

Losing body fat is a very important method of increasing testosterone production. The simple reasoning behind this is that fat deposits increase your body's production of estrogen, which is responsible for decreasing the production of testosterone. So, what basically is happening is that as you accumulate fat, your body produces more estrogen and less testosterone which, in turn allows the body to accumulate more fat. You can stop this vicious cycle by regularly performing cardiovascular workouts, such as running, swimming and rowing. These types of exercises will help to reduce your body fat and keep yourself from accumulating more body fat. 20 minutes a day of cardiovascular workouts will greatly decrease accumulated body fat, especially when coupled with a low fat, high fiber diet.

You should also consider muscle building exercises, such as working with weights or elastic bands. Research has shown that your testosterone level is highest after resistance exercises. The greater the resistance the higher the level of testosterone. Basically this increase of testosterone is affected by the amount of muscle mass being stimulated and the level of intensity. It has also been found that the more muscles being stimulated simultaneously, the greater the amount of testosterone produced. What this boils down to is that multi-joint exercises will stimulate the greatest amount of testosterone (compared to single joint movements). Squats, deadlifts, bench presses, and Olympic lifts are the ideal weight lifting exercises to increase testosterone.

While you may have heard that working out with lighter weights and more reps helps you to prolong your muscular endurance, if your goal is to raise your testosterone level, this method will do very little to help you reach that goal. If you want to release the greatest amount of testosterone, you will want to lift heavier weights, performing only 4 to 5 reps. You will want to lift about 85-

9o% of your 1RM (RM=repetition maximum). If you are fairly new to weightlifting, you might want to start your exercises on weight training machines. After you have built your strength and skill up, you can move on to free weights such as barbells or dumbbells.

One other thing to keep in mind while working out with weights is to use long rest periods between reps. A good rule of thumb is to rest for about 3 minutes between each weight lifting exercise. This doesn't necessarily mean you should just sit on your butt for those three minutes. A good way of resting between reps is by taking this time to stretch, or even doing light calisthenics and working on separate muscle groups.

You should be doing at least 2 to 3 workouts a week in order to obtain maximum testosterone boost. If you are able, I would suggest you find a good personal trainer, as he or she can help you in finding the best workout routines. You might also think about incorporating forced reps into your routine, as well. Forced reps are basically doing as many reps as you are able to, and then forcing yourself to do more reps (with the help of a spotter).

Reducing Stress

While getting the proper amount of sleep and exercise is important in the production of testosterone, one of the best ways of boosting your testosterone level is by reducing stress. When you are under stress your body produces high levels of a hormone called cortisol. The problem is that high levels of cortisol effectively shuts down your body's production of testosterone. If you are under constant stress your body will continuously produce this hormone, which makes it nearly impossible to produce testosterone.

Cortisol production, in and of itself is not necessarily a bad thing. This powerful hormone is produced by your adrenal glands and helps in regulating your blood pressure and immune system, especially in a crises. Cortisol helps by increasing your energy levels and even is helpful in fighting off infections. Therefore a baseline of cortisol is absolutely essential. However, when your body is continuously producing this hormone, it cannot only affect your testosterone production, but also can cause sleep problems , cause spikes and drops in blood sugar levels, and can even cause weight gain. All of these contribute further to decreased production of testosterone.

In today's fast-paced society it is nearly impossible to avoid stress. There is stress on the job, stress at home, stress from social situations, even turning on the news can often increase your stress levels! While you may not be able to avoid stress, luckily there are many ways you can reduce the effects of stress in your life.

<u>Breathing techniques</u>

In high stress situations such as work related stress (boss yelling at you, workload impossible, etc.), deep breathing exercises have been shown to be effective in lowering your body's natural response to stress (the increase of cortisol). The great thing about breathing exercises is that you can do them anywhere at any time, even (and especially) during high stress moments.

The most basic deep breathing exercise (or technique) you can do is simply taking slow deep breaths through your nose and then slowly exhaling out your mouth. The trick is to take as deep a breath as is comfortably possible, hold it for a couple of seconds, and then SLOWLY release the breath, through your mouth. Repeat this a few times and you will find that after a while you will feel much more calm, your blood pressure will decrease, your heart rate will go down, and most importantly, the cortisol levels will return to normal.

Another popular breathing technique is known as the 4-7-8 (or Relaxing Breath) exercise. The 4-7-8 breathing technique was made popular by Dr. Andrew Weil, who says that it is "...utterly simple, takes almost no time, requires no equipment and can be done anywhere"

To perform the 4-7-8 technique you will start out by exhaling through your mouth. Try to exhale as much air as you can while making a "whoosh" sound. Now close your mouth and inhale through your nose, while counting in your head to four. Hold your breath to the mental count of seven, then exhale again through your mouth while making the whooshing sound to the count of eight. Then inhale again through your nose or four seconds, and continue this three times (total of four breaths). You should then breathe normally for a few minutes. If you still feel anxious or stressed, try doing another round of 4-7-8, until you feel the stress released. This is also a great technique to do before bedtime to help you fall asleep, if you have trouble falling asleep or sleeping through the night. One thing to remember when you do this is that the tip of the tongue should remain in the same place throughout the exercise.

The reason the 4-7-8 technique works so well, according to Dr. Weil, is due to the extra oxygen filling the lungs. This extra oxygen has a relaxing effect on the parasympathetic nervous system, which equates to a calming sensation throughout the mind and body. According to Dr. weil, this also helps you to "connect" to your body, giving you a feeling of disconnection from the thoughts and distractions that are causing your sense of anxiety.

Prayer and Spirituality

The last thing you may be thinking of when you are stressed out on your job or in your homelife is that you need to pray more, but a growing number of studies have shown that prayer and spirituality are among the highest ranking stress relievers available to the average person feeling overworked and suffering from high anxiety. Research has shown time and again that people who are more spiritual seem better able to cope with stress, have a quicker healing time from sickness and are (on the average) more healthy than those with no spirituality.

Psychologically speaking, spirituality helps you by allowing you to connect to your world; it allows you to stop trying to be in control of everything... allowing yourself to control what you are able to control and give control over to a higher being or purpose when you feel "out of control". When you realize you are a part of something greater than yourself, you realize you are not responsible for everything that happens in your life, and this gives many people a sense of relief.

According to a study conducted by the National Institute for HealthCare Research (NIHR), college students who were involved in campus ministries actually had less doctor visits and experienced significantly less stress during normally stressful situations than students who had no connections with their campus ministries. Students having strong religious correlations were shown to have much less stress levels and much lower levels of depression and anxiety. To put it succinctly, those students who were religiously involved were better equipped to deal with stress.

Spirituality seems to be a key point in helping one to become less focused on those things that cause stress, such as work deadlines, financial problems, marital problems, etc. This is not to say that those things don't still play an important role in your life, but rather that one is able to see those things with a clear mind, without the stress hormone clouding your judgement and creating more problems than are solved.

By spirituality I am basically talking about something that gives your life meaning or purpose. This could be a set of values or principles, a belief in a higher power or purpose and/or a recognition that there are things outside or beyond the natural world and natural laws governing our lives.

If you are atheistic or agnostic, I am not saying you need to become religious, or start attending Sunday Mass in order to benefit from spirituality. You need not really change any belief system, in order to take advantage of prayer and meditation. While it helps to have a religious belief, or a belief in a higher power, it's not really necessary in order to for "prayer" and meditation to be effective.

One of the reasons why prayer may be so effective is due to the unconscious mind's ability to solve problems that the conscious mind may not be able to solve. For instance, if you are stressed over a work deadline that seems impossible to make, by quieting your mind and focusing on the results you want to achieve rather than the means by which you are going to accomplish them, you may find the answer to the problem that has alluded you. Rather than relying on your conscious mind, which is already stressed and just going around in circles, you allow your unconscious mind to explore possibilities you may not have normally thought of.

The unconscious mind is also capable of controlling things such as blood pressure, heart rate, even body temperature and is even capable of controlling the elevated levels of cortisol in your body, thus reducing your stress and allowing you to concentrate and focus. So whether you are praying to a higher power, or simply talking things over to yourself (either out loud or inwardly), you may find your stress is reduced dramatically and your ability to cope with situations equally improved dramatically.

The infamous A.A. "Prayer of Serenity" is a very good example of how prayer can be used to release tension and improve one's ability to cope with stressful situations. The origins of this prayer are quite hard to verify, though many attribute this prayer to the theologian Dr. Rheinhold Niebuhr, who has told many interviewers that he had written the prayer as part of a sermon delivered on Practical Christianity. Dr. Niebuhr, it must be pointed out, has also been noted as saying that this prayer "may have been spooking around for years, even centuries, but I don't think so. I honestly do believe that I wrote it myself."

Regardless of the origins of the prayer, it has helped hundreds, possibly thousands to cope with, not only the stresses of freeing themselves from alcoholism, but to freeing themselves from stress in general. The prayer (in case you don't know it) goes, "**God grant me the serenity to accept the things I cannot change; the courage to change the things I can; and the wisdom to know the difference.**"

While on the surface this prayer may seem almost too simple, by meditating on this particular prayer you allow yourself to not only free yourself of those things beyond your control, but also encourage yourself to change those things that are within your control. Of course, knowing the difference is the key component. This prayer, said quietly (and possibly repeatedly) will focus your mind and help to reduce your stress.

Also, simply explaining the problems you are facing, the dreams you may have, the struggles you may be going through, will help you to prioritize and bring order to what may seem a confusing and muddled mess. While it helps to have a higher power to focus your prayers to, even the simple act of talking about these things can often help lower stress and bring oneself more into focus. An example prayer might be:

"My life seems out of control, Lord. I cannot seem to do anything right. Help me to be able to see your plan, to understand the purpose in this life. Help me to put my life more on track, and to be able to overcome those numerous obstacles in my way. Help me to get that report I have been trying to write, written. And help me to be a better husband to my wife and better father to my children…" etc.

While you may not use the word "Lord" and, of course, your problems are probably more specific or different, the basic outline of the prayer is the same. Simple speak those things you are having trouble with and then ask for help in overcoming specific areas you feel you need help in. Again, if you ARE religious, you would definitely want to direct those prayers to the object of your faith, but if you are not religious, you can simply direct them to your "inner self" or simple say "I need to focus on such and such, and I want to be better at such and such" etc. So, whether you are religious or not, you can use "prayer" to help you in relieving stress as well as bringing into focus things you can do to improve your daily life.

Meditation

Prayer and meditation often go hand in hand. As a matter of fact, some of the same results seen through prayer can also be observed by regularly meditation. And both prayer and meditation have been practiced for thousands of years. Originally mediation was seen as a means for deepening man's understanding of the spiritual, sacred and mystical forces that rule our lives. However, modern meditation techniques are commonly used as a means for simply relaxing one's body and reducing one's stress. Allowing us to produce within ourselves a sense of tranquility and peacefulness.

Like prayer, one can use meditation as a means of focusing the mind and allowing the jumbled confusions of one's conscious mind to find order and clarity, thus releasing stress and encouraging physical, emotional and psychological well-being. Meditation helps you to clear away all of the garbage that keeps you from seeing clearly and that tends to increase stress, thereby elevating the cortisol levels in your body.

Much like prayer and spirituality, the ability to meditate will often help you to see a new perspective on problems that may be inducing stress on your day to day life. It can help you in building new ways of dealing with those problems by increasing not only your own self awareness, but increasing your awareness of what is happening around you. Meditating also helps you to focus on the here and now, instead of worrying about the future or fretting over past mistakes.

There are many different forms of meditation such as:

- Guided Meditation

- Mindfulness Meditation

- Mantra Meditation

- Transcendental Meditation

- Qi gong

- Tai Chi

And other types of meditations, both ancient and modern. As well as different forms and methods of these meditation. It is well beyond the scope of this book to actually teac you all of the types and forms of meditation available or explain how to perform such meditations, but a basic understanding of some of these meditations can be very beneficial in reducing your stress and keeping your body and mind functioning in harmony.

For instance, in guided meditation, you allow yourself to visualize a place or situation that brings you relaxing. Your guide or teacher will try to bring your visualization into focus, making it seem as real as possible, by incorporating all of your sense, such as smell, sights, sounds, textures, etc. Through this form of meditation you will be able to bring your mind into a place of tranquility, in order to produce a sense of wellness, and peace, thus reducing your stress and improving your cognition. Once you have experienced a few sessions of guided meditations, you will find that you can bring yourself to this peaceful place by yourself in times of increased stress, and almost immediately shut down the cortisol production before it ever gets to an elevated state.

In Mantra Meditations you allow your mind to focus on a simple word or sound (or sometimes a phrase), spoken over and over, until distracting thoughts that are causing the stress are all but eliminated, thus allowing your mind to come into a more focused state. Whereas in Mindful meditation you allow yourself to be more mindful of your own thoughts, by simply allowing yourself to experience the present. You observe thoughts and emotions with a sense of detachment, by simply allowing them to pass without judgement or objectivity.

Other forms of meditation focus on breathing exercises as well as physical movements and such, in order to enhance your own mind and bring yourself into focus. Qi gong and Tai chi are both examples of these type of meditation techniques, where Qi gong in generally about breathing and relaxing movements, and Tai Chi is a form of martial arts, using postures and movements as well as breathing techniques to obtain a sort of oneness of body and mind.

Transcendental meditation is perhaps one of the best known meditation techniques, as it has achieved quite a following in modern times. Transcendental meditation is based on the Vedic tradition of India and was brought to the western world by the late Mharishi Mehesh Yogi in the 1960's. A person practicing transcendental meditation sits in a comfortable position with his or her eyes closed, and repeats a mantra, which is usually given to the person by his or her instructor. This mantry usually is simply a sound, without any sort of meaning. The person then allows their mind to "transcend" thinking, and go into a deeper state of "non thinking" or "pure consciousness. When done properly, a person who practices transcendental meditation achieves a state of peace and tranquility, a sort of stillness where the mind is at rest and sense of order and completeness is experienced. It has been shown through numerous studies that Transcendental Meditation is able to lower the blood pressure, heart rate, and (especially) lower stress hormones (such as cortisol).

Most meditation techniques are simply different forms of the above techniques, with possible additions such as focusing on a certain image or sound, or listening to a certain type of music (or chants). As I said, however, it is really beyond the scope of this book to really teach all the ins and outs of the different meditation techniques, but I would highly recomend anyone interested in easily lowering their stress and increasing self awareness to look into the different meditation techniques outlined here to find one that's right for you!

Laughter Therapy

Perhaps you have heard the expression "laughter's the best medicine"? Well, there is quite a bit of truth to this cliche'd expression. As a matter of fact there have been numerous studies done that show that laughter has a plethora of healthful benefits, including:

1. Boosting the immunity

2. Decreasing Pain

3. Preventing Heart Disease

4. Easing Anxiety

5. Improving Depression

6. Relaxing the Muscles

7. Relieving Stress and Lowering Cortisol

The act of laughing simply makes you feel good, and not only while you are laughing, but even long after your laughter subsides.

It has been shown that laughter actually releases endorphins, those chemicals released by your body that make you feel good. A good hearty laugh is often just as beneficial (if not more beneficial) than almost any drug the doctor could prescribe for stress or anxiety, with absolutely none of the harmfull side-effects.

There are many different ways you can produce this endorphin enhancing, stress reducing, healthy laughter that lightens your mood and increases your happiness and ability to deal with all the negative emotions life seems to induce. Some of the ways you can find to laugh:

• Watch a funny movie or sitcom

• Enjoy some stand up comedy (on TV or a comedy club)

• Find funny people and make them part of your inner circle

• Find good jokes and share them with others

• Go to your library and browse the humor section

• Play with your kids (or your neighbor's kids)

• Allow yourself to be goofy and do something silly

• Go online and search for sites devoted to humor

Also, remember that shared laughter is usually the most effective laughter. Laughter is contagious and often just the sound of one person's laughter can make another person laugh and that person can increase the laughter of the first person, in a sort of humorous domino effect.

Often one of the greatest factors for stress is a lack of humor. A person who takes life too seriously will find that stress is a constant companion. Often, simply finding the humor in situations that may be stressful can alleviate not only your own stress but other's as well. Sometimes it's just a good idea to laugh at life, instead of feeling dread or apprehension.

If you don't find yourself laughing at least a few times a day, you should really try to change this, by being more spontaneous and being less defensive about other people's opinions, judgements or criticism. Also, while a certain amount of inhibition is necessary to exist in society, sometimes letting go of your inhibitions can help you to loosen up and start enjoying life more. Don't be afraid to laugh, not only at circumstances and others, but try to laugh at yourself. After all, we all do crazy things, we all make idiotic mistakes now and then, and we should allow ourselves to laugh at ourselves! This may be one of the easiest (as well as the funnest) ways to lower our stress and to increase our health!

Yoga

Yoga is, in a sense, another type of meditation. However Yoga goes far beyond conventional meditation techniques. The word "yoga" actually means "union", which is to say the union of individual consciousness with the universal conscious or spirit. There are many misconceptions of yoga, such as that yoga is simply about different postures or exercises. While the asanas (or postures) are a part of yoga, they are only a very small part of what yoga is about.

There are actually many different "paths" of Yoga leading toward a goal of self-awareness as the self relates to the whole of the universe... that is to say, becoming one with all that is part of what we call "reality". It is very hard to explain this mindset, especially to the western mind, as this is seen as esoteric; or a spiritual; or transcendent mystical thing. However, part of the goal of Yoga is to actualize that mindset; to understand that which seems incomprehensible, in a clear manner.

The paths toward that goal are seen in the various branches of yoga which includes:

Hatha Yoga -

This branch of Yoga deals with the different physical postures (or asanas). The purpose of the asanas is to purify the body in order to gain a greater awareness of one's self and a greater control over the inner states of the body, which helps to prepare the body for for meditation.

Karma Yoga -

This branch of Yoga is concerned with service to others, in order to enhance the function of the higher or larger self. This is done without thought of the lesser self, such as expecting compensation or even the acknowledgement of self as doer (where the higher self, or God is seen as the ultimate doer). It is a means by which we can achieve a state of peace with even those circumstances that seem insurmountable, or those things that cause undue stress, by experiencing the pure joy of being the instrument by which goodness is manifested.

Mantra Yoga -

As mentioned above, with regards to meditation, a mantra is a certain word or sound repeated in order to focus our minds. Unlike the mantras used in transcendental and other mantra based meditations, in this branch of Yoga, the mantra used are universal root-word sounds, each one representing different aspects of Spirit.

Bhakti Yoga -

This branch of Yoga is a little more difficult to translate or understand. It is basically the surrendering devotion to loving the divinity of all creatures and the "Godness" in everything. This is basically an unending worship of all things created, and by virtue a love of the creator of all things.

Jnana Yoga -

This is the path of wisdom. An explanation of this branch of Yoga is really self-defeating, but suffice it to say that through Jnana (or Gyana) one applies a discriminating intelligence in order to achieve a spiritual liberation.

Raja Yoga -

The Royal Yoga is the highest branch (or path) of Yoga. This can be explored in the Bhagavad Gita and was systematized by Patanjali around 200 BC. This basically combines the essence of all paths of Yoga, by balancing and unifying each approach.

This is a very basic and quite crude explanation of the paths of Yoga, which are subject to interpretation as well as ridicule, but it is difficult to try to present these paths in a way that someone not familiar with yoga can appreciate or understand. However, it is not my intention here to teach the reader about yoga, but rather to express to the reader the greater intricacies of Yoga. That is, to enlighten the reader to understand that yoga is much more than strange postures and breathing techniques.

I, personally, feel that Yoga is the best path for obtaining a stress-free existence. It is, however, not something that can be simply explained or discovered through a book, nor is it is a simple discipline that can be learned overnight. It is a life changing path, that completely changes the way you think and react to life. However, by exploring this particular "discipline" you CAN obtain the ability to not only overcome stress (or obliterate it), but to also achieve health and vitality (both mentally and physically) perhaps unsurpassed by any other means known to man.

You may have noticed that, of the three major ways listed here to increase testosterone production, more attention has been spent on stress than on exercise and sleep. The truth is, both exercise and sleep also help to decrease stress as well, and it might be argued that stress is the most important factor in testosterone production. Of course, stress reduction, alone, isn't going to improve your testosterone production, as it is vital to exercise and get enough sleep as well, but on the whole, reducing your stress is key in increasing your testosterone.

Another contributing factor that we will take up in the next chapter is your diet. What you eat can have a significant impact on your body's ability to produce testosterone. Not only what you eat, but what you don't eat as well. Your diet can also affect other hormonal production in your body and can help regulate production of stress induced hormones. Taken as a whole, increasing testosterone is dependent on diet, exercise, rest (sleep) and stress. By getting the proper amount of sleep, the proper amount of exercise, minimizing stress and eating the right food, you are almost guaranteed a healthy level of testosterone. Not to mention, an increase in vitality and overall health.

CHAPTER 4: TESTOSTERONE LEVELS, WEIGHT LOSS & DIET

As we discussed earlier, your testosterone levels have a great impact on your weight loss goals. More precisely, testosterone has a great impact on your body fat and keeping a good ratio of body fat to muscle. With this in mind, you must be made aware that the traditional weight loss diets actually have a detrimental affect on our testosterone levels, in that most "diets" actually lower your testosterone levels (and quite dramatically).

The reason why traditional weight loss diets have such a dramatic impact on your testosterone levels is because most diets emphasize eating more low-fat foods. However, studies have shown consistently that low-fat high-fiber diets actually lower testosterone levels dramatically, especially if the diet involves eating more polyunsaturated fats.

While I know this goes against what many of you have heard about losing weight, it has been shown time and again that saturated fats and monounsaturated fats are essential in the production of testosterone. What this means is that if you are looking to boost your testosterone level, it's essential that you stay away from any low-fat diets.

For those who are confused on which fats are which here's a breakdown:

• Polyunsaturated fatty-acids (PUFAs) - These are the omega fatty-acids, such as you get from from sunflower oil, safflower oil, flaxseed oil, margarine and light spreads, walnut oil, soybean oil, etc.

- Monounsaturated fatty-acids (MUFAs) - These are obtained through Olive oil, Macadamia Nuts, Sesame Oil, Avocados, Rapeseed oil, Lard, Almonds, etc.

- Saturated fatty-acids (SFAs) - Obtained through Coconut cream, Butter, Suet, Fried Bacon, Cream Cheese, etc.

Scientific studies on the correlation of fat to testosterone levels found that diets higher in saturated and monounsaturated fats significantly increase the levels of testosterone in the body, where diets high in protein and polyunsaturated fats actually reduced the testosterone in the body. These studies also found that the higher the intake of dietary fat (both Monounsaturated and saturated) the higher the testosterone levels seem to be.

It seems, according to these studies that you should derive around 35% to 40% of your daily caloric intake from Saturated Fats and Monounsaturated fats, in order to maintain a healthy testosterone level in your body. You should also try to avoid trans-fats and most Polyunsaturated fatty-acids. However, there is a caveat to the polyunsaturated fats, in that polyunsaturated Omega-3 fatty acids have actually been shown to have a positive impact on testosterone production. These Omega-3 fatty acids are found most abundantly in flaxseeds, walnuts, sardines, salmon, soybeans, brussel sprouts, cauliflower, tofu, shrimp and beef.

The polyunsaturated omega-6 fatty acids are the ones we should actually reduce as much as possible! These fatty acids actually inhibit the production of testosterone, though small amounts of omega-6 fatty acids are essential in our diet. We should try to get most of polyunsaturated fats through omega-3, and less from omega-6 which is contained in many cooking oils (safflower and vegetable oils contain high levels of polyunsaturated omega-6). Mayonnaise is another food that is extremely high in polyunsaturated omega-6 fatty acids and should be avoided at all costs as well as most margarines.

What this basically boils down to is that you a diet that is high in monounsaturated fats, with a bit of saturated fats,some omega-3 polyunsaturated fats and a smidgen of the omega-6 polyunsaturated fatty acids. In order to boost your testosterone, you will want the largest concentration of fats to be of the monounsaturated fats.

I am sure you have probably heard that fat is simply not good for you and you should avoid it, as well as cholesterol being bad for you (well bad cholesterol at least), and so you may be under the impression that this "diet" of fats would be bad for you. While an extreme amount of fats in your diet can, indeed, have a detrimental effect on your health, the truth is that a diet rich in these fats actually does your body good. As well, even cholesterol is beneficial, as long as you do not overdo it. Of course you will want to consult with your doctor if you have cholesterol or heart problems before making any major changes in your diet.

There are also many foods that are known to help in either the synthesis of testosterone, or in lowering (or inhibiting) the production of estrogen. We will discuss a few of these here, and I'll try to give you a brief explanation why each of these foods are helpful in maintaining a good testosterone level. It should be noted, also, that you MUST maintain a good exercise program (explained in the preceding chapter) in conjunction with your diet in order to gain the maximum benefit.

One vegetable that many people tend to avoid in their diet is Brussel Sprouts. This is unfortunate as it is one of the best sources for a compound called I3C (Indole-3-carbinol). I3C helps in boosting your testosterone levels by reducing the aromatase effect, which is when free testosterone is changed into estrogen. As noted earlier, estrogen tends to lower your testosterone levels, so reducing the level of estrogen plays a very important role in raising testosterone levels.

As a matter of fact, studies have found that including a high level of I3C in your diet can help to reduce estrogen by 40% or more, which has a major effect on raising your testosterone levels. If you simply cannot stomach Brussel Sprouts, there are actually quite a few other cruciferous vegetables that contain a good amount of I3C including Garden Cress, Mustard Greens, Kale, Spinach, Broccoli and Cauliflower. If you add one or two servings of these types of vegetables to your diet every day, you can increase testosterone dramatically by decreasing the estrogen being produced in your body.

Another food that has been very helpful in reducing your estrogen levels AND increasing your testosterone levels is blueberries. Blueberries are high in Resveratrol and Calcium-D- Glucarate. Resveratrol has been noted to dramatically reduce estrogen while Calcium-D-Glucarate helps to increase testosterone production. Another food that helps to reduce cortisol is garlic which contains allicin and quercitin, both of which have been shown to inhibit cortisol production.

There have been some that claim that the Bromelain enzyme such as found in pineapples and bananas also help to increase testosterone, but there is actually no evidence to this conclusion. However, it has been shown that fruits high in Vitamin C helps to reduce levels of cortisol which DOES affect testosterone production. It has been long known that eating pineapples, bananas, strawberries, and the like, especially before and after strenuous testosterone building workouts help to keep cortisol at a minimum, in which case testosterone production can be produced at a much more rapid pace and to a much greater degree.

There is some speculation about the aphrodisiac properties of oysters, and the jury is still out on whether or not this is true. However, one thing that is factual is that oysters are extremely beneficial in helping to raise your testosterone levels. The reason for this is mostly due to the high content of Zinc, which has been shown to be a key element in the production of testosterone. A small serving (around 3oz) of oysters contain about 500% of the recommended daily allowance of Zinc. Most beans also contain high levels of Zinc as well as Iron, both of which help in the production of testosterone, and are also packed with more protein than any other plant based food.

Salmon is another food that dramatically increases your testosterone production. This is because Salmon not only contains Omega-3 and high levels of protein (both of which are helpful in testosterone production) but Salmon is also a rich source of Vitamin D, which has also been shown to play a key role in keeping testosterone levels at their peak level!

Eggs have been shown to be an excellent source of cholesterol, which is a key ingredient in increasing your production of testosterone. You may have heard that eggs (because of this cholesterol) were not good for you, but there have been many studies and continuing research that shows this is simply not true. Not only do eggs contain a healthy dose of cholesterol but egg yolks are also a good source of vitamins, minerals and proteins that help your body stay fit and help to increase your testosterone production.

Of course, a good dose of healthy beef is also a great source of Zinc, Proteins and fatty acids, which (as you should be aware of by now) all play a key rolls testosterone production. Pumpkin seeds have also been found to have these key nutrients as well!

While this isn't anywhere near a complete list of dietary foods that will help you in your goal of increasing production of testosterone and inhibiting the production of cortisol and estrogen, it's a great place to start. These are actually amongst the top foods you can consume (and can, indeed, be incorporated into a regular diet quite easily). But it is important to remember, along with a good amount of Zinc, Vitamin D, Protein and other key nutrients, it is important to get your Saturated fats and you monounsaturated fats and (to a lesser degree) polyunsaturated omega-3 and omega-6 fatty acids.

It's important to remember that our glands require zinc and magnesium to get testosterone production started and our Leydig cells require cholesterol in order to continue to produce testosterone. We also need foods high in I3C to boost our testosterone levels by reducing the estrogen level in our body.

One of my favorite breakfasts is bacon and eggs. Which is a very good booster of testosterone, especially when paired with healthy orange (or other fruit) juice and a side of whole wheat toast with butter. I know you may be thinking, THIS IS CRAZY! But, believe it or not, this type of breakfast is packed with what you need to help keep your testosterone flowing at peak levels!

For lunch try incorporating some kale, spinach or a good spring salad mix with some nuts, avocados or olives, and some beef (I prefer some cut up steak), possibly topped with a nice olive oil dressing, and seasoned to taste. This is a great salad mix, not only taste wise but it also packs a plethora of testosterone building vitamins, minerals and essential fats!

Of course, this is just a couple suggestions and for supper you can pretty much eat what you want, just as long as you don't overeat. Eat until you feel full and try to incorporate vegetables and protein, along with a good portion of fats and such in your diet. It's a good idea to have a salad with your meals as often as you can, as well, to add a good portion of necessary vitamins and enzymes. But it's really that simple!

You may be thinking this type of diet will increase your cholesterol levels and make you a prime candidate for a heart attack, but for most people the opposite is true. In most cases this diet will keep your total cholesterol/HDL ratio, LDL/HDL Ratio and Triglycerides/HDL Ratio will at optimal level. Of course, this is contrary to what many doctors may tell you, and what you may have heard or read in many health magazines, but many health professionals are just now realizing how beneficial cholesterol and fatty acids are to our diets and that a small amount of cholesterol in our diets will not increase our overall cholesterol ratios in any negative way whatsoever, but it will help increase our fat burning, health inducing, muscle building testosterone in quite dramatic ways.

CHAPTER 5: BRINGING IT ALL TOGETHER

I need to bring it home that simply changing your diet will not really increase your testosterone to any great degree, nor will simply exercising or getting the proper amount of sleep or reducing your stress levels. At least not individually, but when you combine all of these key components, you will find that not only will you increase testosterone production but you will feel much more energetic throughout the day, your overall health with dramatically improve and your sex life will be out of this world!

While this book is primarily concerned with raising your testosterone levels, you'll find that by putting these principles into motion, you will increase much more than mere testosterone levels. You will increase your longevity, you will increase your vitality, you will increase your very quality of life, and you will be much happier and much more at peace with your own body and mind than you may have ever thought possible.

It will probably be pointed out to me by some that there is much more I could have put in this book, regarding the mechanics of hormones, how testosterone is produced, etc. I could have also gone quite a bit more in depth on exercise methods, methods of stress reduction and such. However, the truth is… everything you need to know about testosterone is written in this book and if this book were much larger, you would probably get lost in the details and quite possible overlook the trees for the forest (so to speak).

So, I have decided to make this book as concise as possible to get you started as quickly and as easily as possible on increasing your testosterone through simple life changes. While these changes are (on the surface) quite simple, they are also quite essential. If you take these methods to heart and actually put them in practice, I can guarantee you that you WILL see a major increase in testosterone and all of the benefits that go along with it.

Another reason I have kept this book as concise as possible is to allow a fairly quick reading, so that you can easily get the gist of what is necessary for you to enhance your testosterone, and you can read it again and again, in order to really grasp the concepts and put them into practice. As I've said in other books I have written, this book is not simply an informational pamphlet to be read and forgotten. This information can not do you any good if you don't actually put it into practice.

If you are thinking it's a little too much to change at one time, then don't change your lifestyle all at once. Work on those things you think you can change easily, such as changing your sleeping habits, lowering your stress levels or possibly instituting an exercise program. Then, when you have successfully managed these components, start slowly instituting other components into your life until you have mastered all of these components. Take your time, but don't put this aside and just think about putting it into practice. If you don't start now, tomorrow may never come. Today is the day to begin changing your lifestyle. If you are (like many men over the age of 40) starting to see that increase in fat around the middle. If you have found your sex drive has been shifted into park. If you find yourself just drudging through the day, with low energy and low vitality, you now have the information to change this. You now know not only what testosterone is and how it affects many aspects of your life, but you are equipped with the knowledge to change this, once and for all.

As I mentioned in an earlier chapter, there are Testosterone Replacement Therapies (Or TRT's) available that will help to increase your testosterone and your doctor may recommend one of these therapies. I am not at all saying that you should not consider TRT, but you may find that these TRT's are only necessary as a stepping stone toward meeting your goal of increasing your testosterone levels and keeping them increased without further need for Testosterone Replacement Therapy.

On the other hand, I would suggest that if you have low sex drive, lack of energy and vitality, low muscle mass and increased fat, then try instituting these changes listed in this book and see where it takes you, you can always go to the doctors and have your Testosterone levels checked, but you may find that you can increase those levels without the need for any kind of injections (or other TRT's), naturally. I can't say whether or not you actually do need therapy to increase your testosterone (and decrease your estrogen and cortisol levels), but it won't hurt to try the natural method first and see where it takes you.

I would also recommend that once you have read this book a couple of times and have a firm understanding of the principles outlined herein, you go ahead and do some more research into the finer points of this book. For instance, go ahead and take some yoga classes, learn some good multipoint resistance exercises or weight lifting exercises. Put together a dietary plan high in the key nutrients and fats listed. Learn of other ways you might increase muscle mass and decrease fat in your body. Go beyond the scope of this book to become an expert in all of the areas outlined herein, until you have become a master of your own body. Don't just read this book and let it end here, let this be your first step toward a journey of lasting health and vitality!

Made in the USA
Middletown, DE
15 November 2022

15084786R00027